# A Simple Guide to
# *Feeding Babies and Toddlers*

Yuchi Yang, MS, RD

**For more information, contact:**
American Nutrition Counseling, LLC
yuchinutrition@yahoo.com
www.anutritioncounseling.com

# Table of Contents

Foreword              i

1    How to Prevent Childhood Obesity              1

2    Benefits of Breastfeeding              12

3    Infant Formula               23

4    Why Eating Solid Foods is More Than Providing Energy and Nutrients              31

5    Dietary Recommendations for Children at Different Developmental Stages              42

6    Building Healthy Eating Habits in Early Childhood Provides Life-Long Benefits              52

Glossary              60

Resources              62

Author              63

Disclaimer              64

# Foreword

I am a pediatric dietitian with more than twenty years of experience working with children, families, and healthcare providers. I am convinced that simple and practical nutrition information can contribute to the well-being of babies and toddlers. I have written this book to help parents by addressing many of their concerns and questions on infant and toddler nutrition.

This book focuses on the following six areas:

1. How to Prevent Childhood Obesity

2. Benefits of Breastfeeding

3. Infant Formula

4. Why Eating Solid Foods is More Than Providing Energy and Nutrients

5. Dietary Recommendations for Children at Different Developmental Stages

6. Building Healthy Eating Habits in Early Childhood Provides Life-Long Benefits

Each chapter starts with some facts and ends with the answers to the most frequently asked questions. In this book, you will find useful information applicable on a daily basis to feed your babies and toddlers.


Yuchi Yang, M.S., R.D.
http://www.anutritioncounseling.com

# Chapter 1

# How to Prevent Childhood Obesity

In this chapter, we shall focus on the root causes of childhood obesity and what we can do to prevent our children from becoming overweight or obese. At the end of this chapter, I also provide the answers to the most frequently asked questions on childhood obesity.

## Causes of Childhood Obesity

Americans are heavier today compared to twenty years ago. One out of every three American adults is obese and 61% are either overweight or obese. Unfortunately, our children are facing the same issues. More than one third of children and adolescents in the U.S. are either overweight or obese.

There are many causes why a lot of American children are overweight or obese:

- Food is more abundant now compared to before. The portion sizes are getting bigger than they were twenty years ago.

- Food companies are adding sugar, salt, fat, and food flavorings to make food more palatable, higher in calories, and readily available. We are exposed to food commercials and vending machines almost everywhere we go.

- American life is getting busier and busier. We spend less time preparing and enjoying food. More often than ever, we are purchasing highly processed food and ready to eat products. Many of these foods are high in sugar, fat, and salt with artificial flavorings.

- Fresh fruits and vegetables may not be readily accessible in some communities. The costs of fresh fruits and vegetables are higher than many high calories and highly processed foods.

- Americans are spending more and more time sitting in front of screens. Based on recent surveys, American adults are spending eight hours every day watching TV, using computer, or playing video games. Children and teens are spending six hours a day in front of a screen.

# Growth Charts for Infants and Children up to 2 Years Old

To find out if your child has a healthy weight, we need to measure it. There are tools to help us to achieve this. The most common used tools are growth charts. Growth charts consist of a series of percentile curves that illustrate the distributions of body measurements in children. There are different growth charts available for infants and children. The World Health Organization (WHO) and the Center for Disease Control and Prevention (CDC) have developed growth charts for parents and doctors to use as tools to monitor children's growth and development. The WHO growth charts are recommended for children under two years of age.

There are two growth charts for children under 2 years of age. One is for boys and the other one is for girls. To find out whether your child has a healthy weight, we use the weight-for-length chart.  Below are the definitions of weight status for children under two years of age:

**Underweight** is defined as a weight-for-length at or under the 5th percentile.

**Normal weight** is defined as a weight-for-length over the 5th and under the 85th percentile.

**Overweight** is defined as a weight-for-length at or above the 85th percentile and lower than the 95th percentile.

**Obesity** is defined as a weight-for-length at or above the 95th percentile. The weight-for-length growth charts for boys and for girls are included in the following as Figure 1-1 and Figure 1-2.

There are three simple steps to find out whether your child (birth to 2 years of age) has a healthy weight. First, you select the right growth chart based on the gender of your child. Second, you simply plot the child's height and weight measurements on the growth chart. Third, compare the plotted dot to the definitions of weight status shown above.

**Figure 1-1: Weight-for-Length Growth Chart: Boys.**

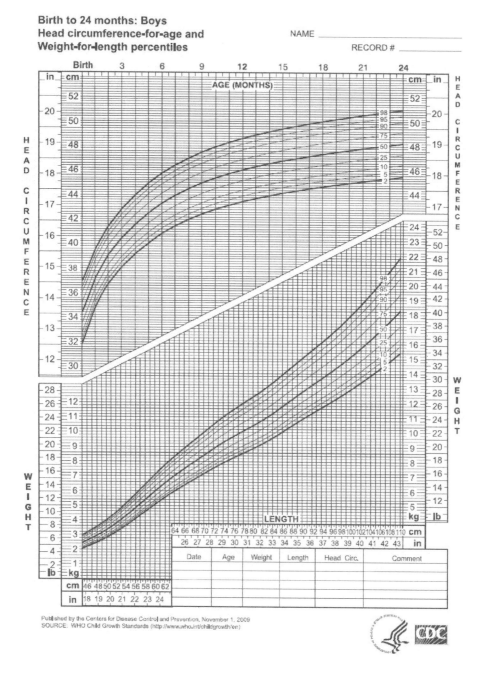

Birth to 24 months: Boys
Head circumference-for-age and
Weight-for-length percentiles

**Figure 1-2: Weight-for-Length Growth Chart: Girls.**

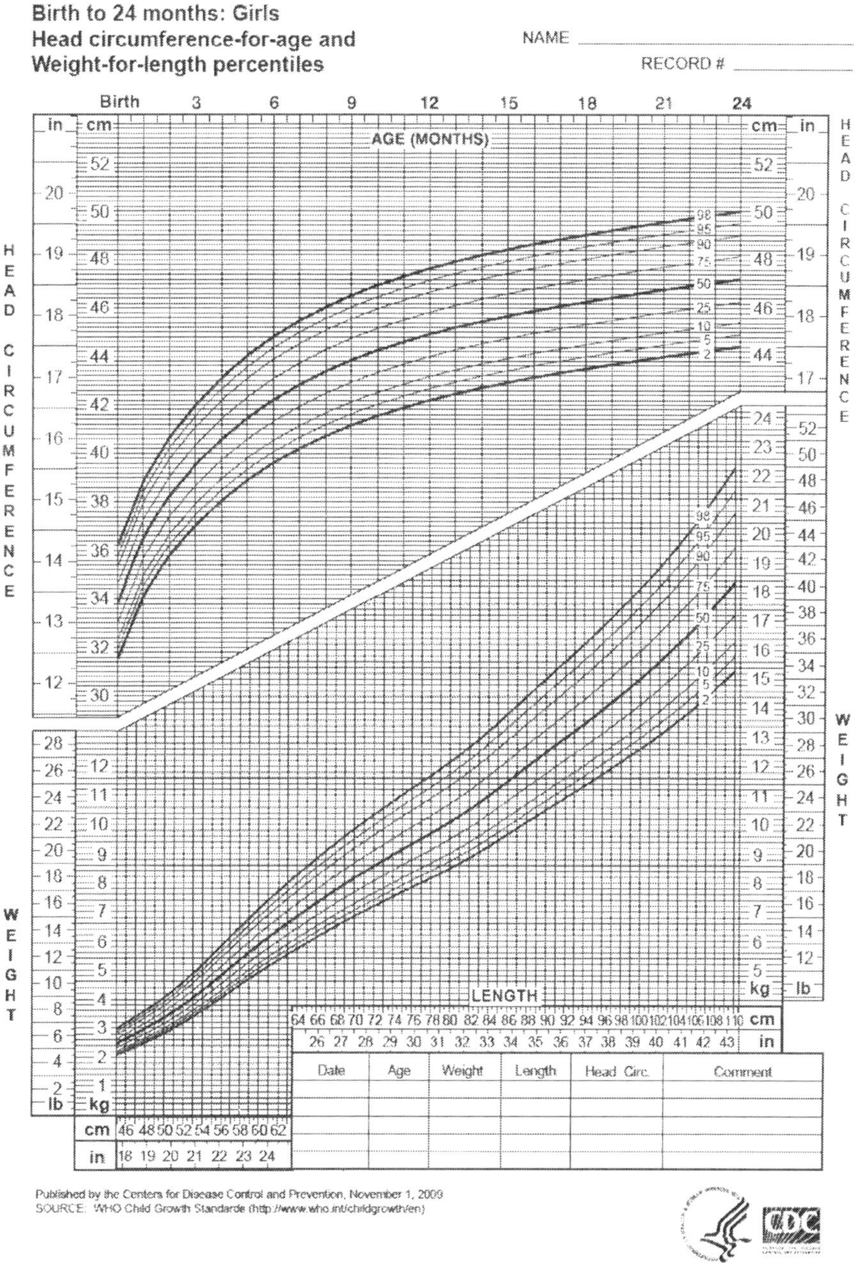
Birth to 24 months: Girls
Head circumference-for-age and
Weight-for-length percentiles
NAME
RECORD #
Birth 3 6 9 12 15 18 21 24
AGE (MONTHS)
HEAD CIRCUMFERENCE
WEIGHT
LENGTH
Date
Age
Weight
Length
Head Circ.
Comment
Published by the Centers for Disease Control and Prevention, November 1, 2009
SOURCE: WHO Child Growth Standards (http://www.who.int/childgrowth/en)

Yuchi Yang, R.D.

As an example for an 18-month old girl weighing 29 pounds and 8 ounces and having a length of 33 inches, when we plot her weight and length measurements on the WHO growth chart, her weight-for-length (the pointer) is over the 95<sup>th</sup> percentile curve. Therefore, she is obese. Below is how her grow chart looks like:

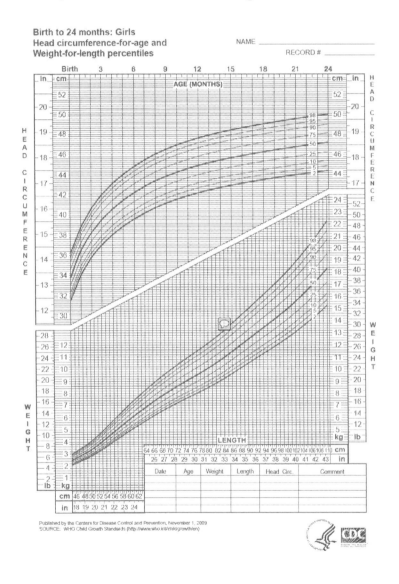

# Body Mass Index for Children Older than Two Years of Age

Body Mass Index (BMI) for most people is a reliable index of body fatness. The BMI is calculated from height and weight. Here is the BMI formula:

Formula: weight (lb) / [height (in)]$^2$ x 703

For children older than two years of age, we use the BMI-for-age percentile to monitor whether the child has a normal weight. Instead of doing your own BMI calculation, you can visit the Center for Disease Control and Prevention (CDC) website: http://apps.nccd.cdc.gov/dnpabmi/. On the web page, you can enter your child's age, gender, height, and weight to get the BMI value and the BMI-for-age percentile. A child's weight status is defined based on the BMI-for-age percentile, not the absolute number of BMI. Here are the definitions of weight status using the BMI-for-age percentiles for children (2–18 years of age):

**Underweight** is defined as a BMI-for-age at or under the 5th percentile.

**Normal weight** is defined as a BMI-for-age over the 5th and under the 85th percentile.

**Overweight** is defined as a BMI-for-age at or above the 85th percentile and lower than the 95th percentile.

**Obesity** is defined as a BMI-for-age at or over the 95th percentile.

For example, for a 3-year-old boy who is 4 feet tall and weighs 50 pound, the report looks like:

*Based on the height and weight entered, the BMI is 15.3, placing the BMI-for-age at the 24th percentile for boys aged 3 years. This child has a healthy weight.*

# Strategies to Help Your Child Build Healthy Eating Habits

- Offer healthy meals and snacks.

- Teach your young children to follow consistent meal times, meal settings, and healthy eating habits. This is a crucial time for young children to begin to use meal time routines and set appropriate expectations.

- Learn your children's cues for hunger and satiety. Offer small amount of food at first; serve a second serving if needed.

- Allow children to explore the food and learn the fine motor skills of feeding themselves. Although this can be a little messy at times, with some preparation prior to the meals, you can decrease the amount of clean-up afterwards. For example, put a newspaper or a cloth underneath your child's chair will make the clean-up easier for you.

- Talk with your child about food choices related to your culture, family choices, and health.

- Some children prefer having a choice of foods. Instead of saying, "Would you like to have an apple?" You might want to say, "Would you like to have an apple or a pear?" When you ask a question like this, young children more likely will pick one of these two choices. Although it is a good idea to offer choices, it may lead to more issues if you offer more than two options.

- Enforce positive behavior by rewarding with attention, not with food. Refrain from using food especially sweets as rewards; celebrate with praises and excitement instead.

- It is fine to serve sweets and treats for special occasions such as birthdays.

Eat with your child. Eating time is for you and your child to relax and enjoy food and quality time together. Kids who have family meals tend to eat healthier foods.

# Frequently Asked Questions and Answers

**Q: My baby (or young child) looks a little bit chubby. What should I do?**

A: Healthy babies and young children come in different sizes and shapes. As parents, we can:

- Be a good role model. Children learn by observing and imitating the adults around them. Parents are the most influencing people in children's lives. Eating healthy as a family will help children establish good eating habits.

- Shop wisely:

    o Shop on the perimeter of the grocery store. Fresh fruits, vegetables, dairy, meats, and grains in most markets are displayed on the perimeter of the market.

    o Read the nutrition fact labels and the ingredient list when you buy packaged food. Avoid foods and beverages that are high in saturated fats, trans fats, added sugars, and sodium (salt).

- Plan meals, snacks, eating schedules, and meal settings ahead of time. Planning meals and snacks can save you time and money. For example, when you go out with your children, bring some healthy snacks with you.

- Have regular meal/snack time schedules.

- Offer water instead of sweet beverages. Limit 100% juice to 4 ounces a day. Americans in general are consuming too much sweet beverages. Sweet beverages are the largest single source of added sugar in the American diet today.

- Offer small servings of food first, if needed, provide a second serving.

- Provide healthy meals and snacks.

- Refrain from using food as rewards for good behaviors, use praise and attention instead.

- Reserve sweets for special occasions like birthdays. Most of us like sweets. Kids are no exceptions. The key is not to eat sweets/deserts frequently. When it is time to enjoy sweets/deserts, pay attention to the amount we are providing to our children.

- Limit screen time. American people are spending many hours in front of a screen such as TV, computers, and video games each day. Studies have shown that children are more active, behave better, and eat healthier when they spend less time in front of a screen.

- Refrain from making negative comments about your child's weight. As parents, we all want the best for our children. Although with good intention, sometimes we are too concerned and may have made some comments that do not help the situation. For example, if a child wants to buy cakes, instead of making negative comments like, "You are too chubby to eat cakes." You may want to tell the child that "We are not buying cakes today because it is not your birthday." A statement like this does not negatively impact the child's feeling about food and his or her body image/weight; it also teaches the child that sweets/deserts are reserved for special occasions or celebrations.

- Redirect the attention of young children from sweets/deserts to somewhere else.

- Encourage your children be physically active. Enjoy play time with your children and engage them in group activities.

Most healthy babies and young children have ability to regulate their food intake over time to get the energy and nutrients they need. There is no need to worry as long as we are offering healthy food to them. Let us allow our children to decide the amount of food that they would like to eat. This will help them to build a healthy relationship with nutritious food. Over time many of them will lose their baby fat when they eat healthy foods and stay physically active.

# Chapter 2

# Benefits of Breastfeeding

In this chapter, we shall cover the benefits of breastfeeding, breastfeeding positions, proper latch-on, nurse on demand, where you can find breastfeeding support, breastfeeding resources, and answers to the frequently asked questions.

**For the past several decades, numerous studies have shown that breastfeeding is the best choice for healthy babies and mothers.**

Breast milk protects babies from illness and provides excellent nutrition for babies' growth and development. Breastfed babies are less likely to develop allergies and overweight problems. In addition, a child's first year is crucial for the brain development and human milk increases babies' Intelligence Quotient (IQ) scores.

Breastfeeding is good for the nursing mothers as well. Nursing moms are less likely to develop breast and ovarian cancer later in their lives. Breastfeeding also helps to create a special bond between the mother and the baby.

More and more mothers in the U.S. are aware of these benefits. Therefore, breastfeeding initiation rate has been increasing steadily. At present, about three out of four mothers in the U.S. initiate breastfeeding; however, less than half of them breastfeed for six months.

Breastfeeding comes naturally and easily for many mothers. Some nursing mothers do experience difficulties and quit nursing earlier than they would like to. Therefore, many government agencies, universities, hospitals, private organizations, and communities are working together to provide necessary support for nursing mothers to continue breastfeeding as long as they choose to.

## Breastfeeding Basics

**Step one: Nursing mothers need to have adequate rest, eat well, and drink plenty of liquids.**

When you are feeling well, you can do a better job of taking care of your baby. Good nutrition and lots of liquids will help nursing mothers produce more milk.

**Step two: Make sure that the nursing position is comfortable for you and your baby.**

You may want to have a nursing pillow or use regular pillows to support nursing positions of your choice. Commonly used positions include:

**Cradle hold – the most popular position**

Cradle hold is like the way you would cradle your baby in your arms, as illustrated here. This is the classic position many mothers would use often at home or outside of the house.

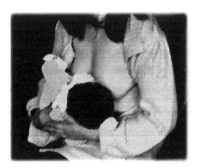

**Football hold**

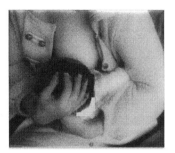

As illustrated above, you tuck your baby under your arm, like a running back holding a football going for a touch-down. You might want to place a pillow on your side to support your baby or your arm to feel more comfortable. You may want to try the football hold when:

- You have had a cesarean section and want to avoid placing your baby against your abdominal incision.

- You would like to see better and make sure that your baby has a perfect latch-on.

- You want to nurse twins simultaneously.

**Lying down – nursing moms using this position can rest while nursing.**

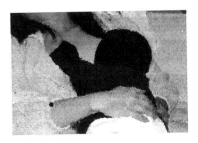

This position can work either lying on your back or on your side. Your baby is facing you, forming a tummy-to-tummy position. This position works well for a mother who is recovering from a cesarean section as the baby is not leaning on the cut. For your baby's safety, you must remain alert and do not fall asleep while nursing the baby using the lying down position.

**Step three: The baby has a correct latch-on.** Latch-on is how your baby put your breast into his or her mouth.

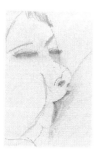

Correct latch-on helps provide you with a painless breastfeeding experience. It helps your baby to express milk from your breast more efficiently. Below are the steps for a correct latch-on:

1. First, make your baby open his or her mouth wide.

2. Gently pull your baby towards your breast. Do not lean forward to your baby.

- With a correct latch-on, the baby's lips turn outward and the mouth is open wide. Almost the entire areola is in your baby's mouth.

- After a few seconds of nursing, your nipple should not feel pain. If you feel pain after few seconds, the latch-on is not correct.

- If the latch-on is not correct, you need to stop and repeat the process. Do not just pull the baby back. This will hurt your nipple. Break the sucking by gently putting one of your fingers into the corner of your baby's mouth. With practice, your baby will learn how to do it right the first time.

### Step four: Begin nursing at a different breast.

Many babies express milk more efficiently at the beginning with stronger sucking. Therefore, it is a good idea to begin a nursing session at a different breast from the previous feeding. For example, if you start nursing on the right breast this time, then you may want to start nursing on the left next. You can use a pin on your shirt to remind yourself which side of the breast you should feed your baby next.

### Step five: Nurse on demand or on cues.

Babies grow rapidly during the first 12 months. They usually double their birth weight by six months and triple their birth weight by 12 months. A newborn baby may nurse as frequently as every two hours since they have tiny stomachs with limited space. When the baby has had enough, usually the baby will let go of your breast. A nursing session takes about 20 - 40 minutes (10 - 20 minutes on each breast). As babies grow bigger and stronger, they may nurse more effectively and a nursing session may be as short as 5 - 10 minutes on each breast.

It is important to nurse on demand or on cues because babies experience several growth spurts during the first year. Every baby's growth pattern is different. Growth spurts usually occur at these ages: 2 - 3 weeks, 6 weeks, 3 months, 6 months, and 9 months. When babies have their growth spurts, they need to be nursed frequently and a nursing session may last for a longer period of time.

Some mothers may become concerned and think that they do not have enough milk for their babies. In fact, it is normal for babies to nurse more frequently and for a longer period of time during their growth spurts. This will enable babies to get the amount of calories and nutrients that they need for their rapid growth. The signs that your baby is going through a growth spurt follow:

- Your baby wants to be breastfed more frequently. Each nursing session takes longer than before. A growth spurt usually lasts only for few days.

- Your breast should feel full or fuller before nursing and feel softer after the feeding.

- Your Baby has more wet diapers within a day.

- The baby is gaining weight. Weight gain is the best indicator that the baby is going through a growth spurt.

## Individuals who provide breastfeeding support:

- **Trained breastfeeding peer counselors** are individuals who are trained to provide assistance and support for some common breastfeeding concerns. Many of them have experiences of nursing their own babies.

- **International Board Certified Lactation Consultants (IBCLCs)** are experts who have specialty trainings in breastfeeding and can help nursing mothers and their babies with more complex problems. Many of them are registered nurses or registered dietitians.

## Resources:

- National Breastfeeding Help line: 800-994-9662.

- La Leche League website: http://www.llli.org/ .

# Frequently Asked Questions and Answers

**Q: How can I connect with other breastfeeding mothers in my community?**

A: Check with your birthing hospital, they may have a breastfeeding support group or classes. You may also find a La Leche League Leader or Group near you by visiting a La Leche League website http://www.llli.org/webus.html.

**Q: How can I find a Lactation Consultant for more help?**

A: To find a Lactation Consultant in your community, ask your baby's doctor. Your baby's doctor may have a list of Lactation Consultants in your area. You can also try to locate a Lactation Consultant by visiting the website of the International Lactation Consultant Association http://www.ilca.org/i4a/pages/index.cfm?pageid=3432.

**Q: Is it normal that my nipples are sore?**

A: Some women experience sore nipples for the first few days of nursing their babies. If your nipples are sore, you need to pay more attention to the nursing position and how the baby latches onto your breast. Make sure the nursing position is correct and the baby has opened the mouth wide enough to get a good grasp onto your breast. With a good latch-on, the baby's nose will touch or get very close to the breast.

Apply small amount of lanolin to the sore nipples. Lanolin is a grease/wax secreted from wool-bearing animals such as sheep. You can find lanolin cream in the aisle of baby or nursing products in a grocery store. Lanolin will help to relieve pain and allows the nipples to heal faster. There is no need to wash off the cream before nursing.

If the nursing position and latch-on are correct, the sore nipple problem should resolve in a few days. If this problem persists, consult a Lactation Consultant for more help.

**Q: I just drank a glass of wine. Can I breastfeed my baby afterward?**

A: Substance like alcohol could pass into breast milk and may be harmful to your baby. Substance abusers should not breastfeed. If you are an occasional drinker and just had a glass of wine, it is a good idea to wait a few hours for your body to clear up the alcohol. Then, pump the breast milk out and discard the milk.

You can resume nursing your baby once alcohol is completely out of your body and after you have pumped and dumped the contaminated milk.

**Q: Is my baby getting enough breast milk?**

A: You can:

- Make sure that the nursing position is comfortable for you and your baby, and the baby has a good latch-on. This allows the baby to suck and swallow the milk more efficiently. The more the baby expresses the milk, the more milk you will produce for the next feeding. After each feeding, your breasts should feel soft.

- Breastfeed frequently. Newborn babies need to be nursed 8-12 times within 24 hours. The more your nurse, the more milk your body will produce.

- Bring your baby to the doctor for regular check-ups. The doctor will monitor baby's length and weight measurements. If your baby has normal growth and weight gain, the baby is getting enough breast milk. Many babies, if not all, lose a small amount of body weight in the first few days and then gain back the weight by the first week or two.

- Count the number of wet diapers that your baby has in 24 hours. If your baby has six or more wet diapers a day, the baby is getting enough.

- Observe the baby. If your baby is content after nursing and is alert, the baby is getting enough breast milk.

If you have concerns, talk to your baby's doctor or a Lactation consultant. To estimate the amount of breast milk that your baby has taken in during a feeding, a Lactation consultant can take your baby's weight before and after a nursing session.

**Q: I am exclusively breastfeeding my baby. Should I give my baby water?**

A: There is usually no need to give your baby water. Breast milk should provide all the liquids your baby needs for the first 4-6 months of life.

If you live in a very hot environment, check with your baby's doctor to see if a small amount of water is needed.

**Q: How long should I breastfeed my baby?**

A: It is recommended that mothers breastfeed their babies exclusively for four to six months. Then introduce solid foods while continue to breastfeed their babies at least through the first year.

**Q: How can I continue breastfeeding after returning to work?**

A: Working mothers can continue to breastfeed by pumping and storing milk when they are away from their babies. There are a variety of breast pumps available in the market.

A more powerful electric breast pump usually works better for maintaining milk supply after returning to work.

Manual pumps and less powerful electric breast pumps are good choices for occasional users or for mothers who have established a good milk production.

It is a good idea to pump and store some breast milk in the freezer several weeks prior to returning to work. This helps nursing mothers get familiar with the pump and make sure that there are enough supplies of breast milk for your baby after you return to work.

Breast milk can be safely stored in a sterile bag for two days in the refrigerator or for two weeks in a freezer compartment located inside a refrigerator or for three months in a freezer with a self-contained door.  Remember to put the date on the bag and always use the oldest milk first.

When you are at home with your baby during evenings and weekends, enjoy nursing your baby. This helps you maintain a good supply of breast milk.

# Chapter 3

# Infant Formulas

In this chapter, we shall cover the different types of formulas in the market, proper ways to warm up the formulas, resources, and answers to the frequently asked questions.

If you choose to bottle feed your baby with a formula, check with your baby's doctor to see which formula is right for your baby. There are many different types of formulas available in the market. Most of the formulas come in different forms such as ready-to-feed, powder, and concentrated cans.

## Types of Formulas

### Milk-based formulas:

Milk-based formulas are the most popular formulas. Many babies drink milk-based formulas without any problems while some babies may need a different formula due to milk allergy, intolerance, and/or medical conditions.

### Partially hydrolyzed formulas:

The Protein in this formula has been partially broken down into smaller parts. It is usually used for babies who cannot tolerate the whole protein in the milk-based formula.

## Soy based formulas:

It is milk-free and lactose-free. Lactose is a sugar found in milk. Some pediatricians recommend soy formulas for babies with milk protein sensitivity or allergy. Soy formulas can also be used for parents who prefer a vegan diet for their babies.

## Therapeutic formulas:

A variety of therapeutic formulas are available for babies with various food allergies, intolerance, and/or medical conditions. For example, babies with metabolic disorders who cannot metabolize certain amino acids should use metabolic formulas.

# Different Forms of Infant Formulas

## Ready-to-feed formulas:

Preparation and feeding: Wash the can before you open it. Pour the right amount into a bottle and feed the baby. Discard the leftovers in the bottle that the baby does not finish.

You can store the remaining formula in the can or pour them into different bottles and store them in the refrigerator up to 48 hours.

## Powder formulas:

Preparation and feeding: Wash the can before you open it. Follow the preparation instructions on the can. Use the scoop provided in the can. When you scoop up the powder, make sure you level the power off. Do not pack down the powder. For standard dilution, put 1 scoop of formula into every 2 ounces of water.

## Concentrated cans:

Preparation and feeding: Wash the can before you open it. Follow the preparation instructions on the can. For standard dilution, mix the concentrated formula with the same amount of water. For example, if you are preparing 4 ounces of formula for your baby, you need to pour 2 ounces of formula from the concentrated can to a bottle and mix it with 2 ounces of water.

Ready-to-feed formula is convenient; however, the cost is higher than the powder and the concentrated cans. After you follow the preparation instructions listed on the can, regardless of which form you use, the same formula yields similar amount of calories and nutrients.

# Ways to Warm Up the Formulas

- Use warm water to mix with formula from the concentrated can or the formula powder.

- Warm a bottle of formula in a pot with hot water.

- Use a bottle warmer.

Do not use microwave to heat up the formula. The temperature can be uneven and the baby may get burned from the formula.

**Always test the temperature of the formula by putting a drop of formula on your inner wrist before feeding the baby.**

# Internets:

- http://www.enfamil.com

- http://www.gerber.com

- http://similac.com/

# Frequently Asked Questions and Answers

**Q: How do I know when my baby is hungry or need something else?**

A: Every baby gives out different cues for hunger. Observe and get to know your baby. Some babies may put fists in their mouths, some may smack lips, some may open their mouths, and some may fuss and start crying. Be patient, over time, you will learn how to read your baby's cues for hunger.

**Q: How do I know when my baby is full?**

A: Every baby is unique. Some may fall asleep when they are full. Some may stop sucking or slow down the pace of sucking. Some may even turn away from the nipple. When your baby is full and loses interest in feeding, it is time to stop even if there is still some formula left in the bottle.

**Q: Can I save any leftover formula that my baby did not finish in a bottle?**

A: No. If your baby does not finish the entire bottle, discard the leftovers. Germs and enzymes from your baby's mouth can spoil it.

**Q: Can I put cereals in a bottle?**

A: No. For healthy babies, it is not recommended to put cereals in a bottle.

- Babies younger than 4 months of age do not need cereals. All they need is breast milk or formula.

- After thickening the formula with cereals, formula may not flow well out of a bottle. For that reason, some parents enlarge the opening of bottle nipple, which is not recommended.

- Putting cereals in a bottle adds extra calories that will put babies at risk of becoming overweight or obese.

**Q: Why do some infant formulas contain probiotics?**

A: Probiotics are live microorganisms beneficial to our body. Breastfed babies have more probiotics found in their stools compared to formula fed babies. Some studies have shown that probiotics help to strengthen babies' developing immune system.

For healthy babies, probiotics supplemented formula are considered safe. However, these formulas should not be given to infants who are chronically or seriously ill.

**Q: Why do some infant formulas contain prebiotics?**

A: Prebiotics are found in human milk. To human bodies, prebiotics are not digestible but they are food to feed probiotics (good bacteria) in our intestines. Studies have shown that prebiotics may improve the health of our gut and bowel movement.

**Q: Why do infant formula companies add DHA and EPA to the infant formula?**

A: Docosahexaenoic acid (DHA) and Arachidonic acid (ARA) are good fats that are naturally present in human milk. Studies have found that DHA and ARA have many health benefits to the baby's brain and eye development.

**Q: When should I introduce cow's milk to my baby?**

A: If a baby has no milk allergy, it is recommended to introduce whole cow's milk at 12 months of age.

**Q: Can I give my 1 year-old child low fat milk?**

A: No. It is recommended to give young children under 2 years of age whole milk, not low fat milk. Children under 2 years of age grow rapidly and they need the fat from the whole milk to meet their nutritional needs.

**Q: My baby is constipated. Can I feed my baby low iron formula?**

A: No. Although some people might believe that iron causes constipation; however, studies have not shown a correlation between the right amount of iron intake and constipation. Besides, iron is an essential nutrient that our bodies need. Without adequate amount of iron, babies will develop iron deficiency anemia.

Regular infant formula provides the right amount of iron that healthy babies need for growth and development. Low iron formula is designed for babies with some rare medical conditions and is not suggested for alleviating constipation.

To alleviate your baby's constipation problem, you can try the following:

- Talk with your baby's doctor. There are many factors that can cause babies being constipated. Your baby's doctor can help figure out the possible causes and come up with a treatment plan.

- Discuss with your baby's doctor to see whether a formula added with prebiotics is right for your baby. Some formula companies have added prebiotics to their starter infant formulas. Babies receiving prebiotics through these formulas tend to have softer and more frequent stools.

- As babies grow, their guts will become stronger and the constipation problem usually improves. When your baby is ready for solid foods, you can offer fruits and vegetables that are high in fiber, for example, apricots, peaches, plums, pears, bananas, strawberries, blueberries, apples, peas, spinach, corn, broccoli, green beans, squash, and carrots. Dietary fibers attract water into the intestines, thus softening the stools. In addition, dietary fibers exercise the intestinal muscles so that the guts retain their health. While increasing dietary fiber, it is important to make sure that your baby gets adequate amount of liquids.

- Introducing yogurts with active culture to older babies (8 months or older) may help to soften their stools and improve bowel movement.

# Chapter 4

## Why Eating Solid Foods is More Than Providing Energy and Nutrients

In this chapter, we shall cover the benefits of eating solid foods, time to start different solid foods, making your own baby foods, buying commercial baby foods, meal time supervision, and answers to the frequently asked questions on how to introduce solid foods.

## Benefits of Eating Solid Food

- Solid foods provide energy and nutrients to meet your babies' growing needs.

- Different solid foods have different colors, smell, and tastes. Eating solid food will provide opportunities for your baby to enjoy and appreciate the experience of eating.

- Eating solid foods allows the babies to develop a variety of fine motor skills. Solid foods come in different sizes, shapes, and textures. With practice, your baby will be able to eat different food textures over time. They will start finger feeding, eat with a spoon, and drink from a cup.

## Time to Start Solid Food

It is recommended to introduce solid foods after four months of age. If you are exclusively breastfeeding your baby, there is no need to start solid food until he or she is six months of age. If your baby drinks infant formula, you can start feeding your baby solid foods when he or she can sit independently or sit with some support and shows interest in solid foods. Most babies reach this developmental milestone before six months of age.

## Time to Start Finger Food

When the babies are capable of picking up food using their thumbs and forefingers and putting food into their mouths, they are ready for finger foods. Soft cooked vegetables, fruits, o-shape cereals, a slice of bread, and crackers are good finger food choices.

## Time to Start a Cup

You could start your baby with a cup when he or she can sit without help, grasp an object with both hands, and bring it to the mouth. These are the fine motor skills needed for drinking from a cup.

## Time to Use a Spoon

Many young children from 12-18 months of age feed themselves with a spoon. Although sometimes it can be quite messy, it is surely fun to watch them learn and master their fine motor skills of self-feeding.

## Making Your Own Baby Foods

Always wash your hands before preparing your own baby foods to protect your baby from food borne illness.

A small food processor (1-3 cups) makes your job easier. You can simply clean and wash fresh fruits and puree them in a small food processor right before the feeding. For some drier or harder fruits, you may consider adding one tablespoon of water when you make pureed baby food. There is no need to add sugar when you make the pureed fruit. The natural taste of fruits is delicious.

You may want to boil or steam vegetables before you put them in the food processor. You can make a larger amount and save them in small containers and store them in the fringe for a couple of days, or in a freezer for a longer period of time.

There is no need to add oil or salt when you make pureed vegetables. The baby's taste bud is quite sensitive and the pure and natural taste of vegetables, for example, carrots, green beans, and peas, is quite yummy.

To prepare pureed meats, for food safety, make sure that the meats are well cooked before you put them in the food processor. Just like vegetables, you can make larger amount and store them in the fringe for a couple of days or in a freezer for a longer period of time.

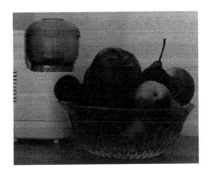

## Buying Baby Foods

When buying baby foods, it is important to read the nutrition fact label. The food label tells us the serving size and the number of servings in a package, the amount of calories and nutrients in a single serving, and the amount of fat, salt, and sugar.

Remember to check the ingredient list. Ingredients are listed in descending order by weight. The ingredients in the larger amounts are listed first. The ingredient list shows us whether or not the product contains added sugar, fat, salt, artificial flavors, preservatives, and others.

If your baby has food allergies, pay close attention to the ingredient list when you buy packaged foods. The U.S. law requires food companies to clearly state if the product contains the eight major allergenic foods. They are milk, eggs, fish, crustacean shellfish, tree nuts, peanuts, wheat, and soybeans. If your baby has food allergies other than these eight foods, consult with a registered dietitian (RD). A dietitian can work with you on how to avoid the offending or allergenic food while making sure that your child is getting the right amount of calories and nutrients from the food he or she eats.

Please find an example of nutrition facts and an ingredient list for a pack of baby organic green beans below:

## Nutrition Facts

Serv. Size 1 pack
Servings Per Container 2 packs

Amount Per Serving

**Calories** 35

| | |
|---|---|
| **Total Fat:** | 0g |
| Trans Fat: | 0g |
| **Sodium:** | 10mg |
| **Potassium:** | 180mg |
| **Total Carbohydrates:** | 8g |
| Fiber: | 2g |
| Sugar: | 3g |
| **Protein:** | 2g |

**%Daily Value**

| | |
|---|---|
| Protein: | 4% |
| Vitamin A: | 15% |
| Vitamin C: | 0% |
| Calcium: | 6% |
| Iron: | 4% |
| Vitamin E: | 30% |
| Zinc: | 4% |

**Ingredients**
ORGANIC GREEN BEANS, WATER, TUNA OIL (SOURCE OF DHA), CHOLINE BITARTRATE, GELATIN, ALPHA TOCOPHERYL ACETATE (VITAMIN E)

## Mealtime Supervision

A lot of choking occurs when children eat while running around. They should be seated during mealtimes. If your child is seated in a high chair, make sure that the safety strap is fastened properly.

Keep sharp utensils out of their reach. Consider using unbreakable plates and cups when they learn how to feed themselves.

Children can be unpredictable especially during mealtimes. Watch over closely when your child eats. This way, you can prevent or quickly respond to unexpected events.

# Frequently Asked Questions and Answers

**Q: What food should I avoid giving to my baby?**

A: These are the general guidelines:

- Do not give honey to babies younger than one year of age. Honey may cause infant botulism, an illness that can be very serious.

- Avoid foods that may be too difficult for a baby to chew or swallow. Food, including nuts, seeds, popcorn, hotdogs, jelly, candies, whole grapes, and peanut butter, can become lodged in a small child's throat and cause choking.

- Avoid egg white and shellfish in the first year. For babies with a family history of food allergies, consult the baby's doctor to see whether you should delay giving these types of food to your baby, including eggs, milk, wheat, peanuts, citrus, and others.

**Q: How do I introduce solid foods?**

A: Many parents start with baby cereals. Mix cereals with formula or breast milk in a bowl and feed them with a soft-tip spoon. If you prefer, you may start with pureed vegetables or fruits. When introducing a new food, wait a few days to make sure that your baby does not develop an allergic reaction to that food before you introduce another one. At the beginning, offer one to two tablespoons. If your baby has no allergic reaction to the food, you can give more the following day.

Usually, meats are introduced last, after baby has been eating cereals, fruits, and vegetables. Some babies may be more willing to try solid foods when they are hungry. Offering solid foods before giving breast milk or formula may also help them accept new food. Another tip is to choose a time that your baby is not tired or cranky.

## Q: What are food allergies?

A: A food allergy is an exaggerated immune response triggered by food. Symptoms range from mild to severe reactions. Severe food allergies can be life-threatening.

There is no cure for food allergy. Strict avoidance of food allergens is the only way to prevent the allergic reactions. More infants and children have food allergies today than before. Children usually outgrow their egg, milk, and soy allergies, but some may have food allergies for life.

The U.S. law identifies the eight most common allergenic foods. These foods account for 90 percent of all food allergies. The U.S. law requires food companies to identify these eight foods on the food labels. They are:

1. Milk

2. Eggs

3. Fish

4. Crustacean shellfish such as crab, shrimp

5. Tree nuts such as almonds, pecans

6. Peanuts

7. Wheat

8. Soybeans.

The following is an example of ingredients listed on a package for "organic fruit yogurt smoothies":

**Ingredients:** Organic Bananas, Organic Peaches, Water, Organic Yogurt (Organic Cultured Pasteurized Milk), Calcium Citrate, Ascorbic Acid (Vitamin C), Citric Acid, Vitamin D. **CONTAINS: MILK.**

By reading the ingredient list for organic fruit yogurt smoothies, we learn that this product is not suitable for children with milk allergy.

For information on the treatment and management plan for food allergies, please talk to your child's doctor.

**Q: Why should my baby drink from a cup?**

A: There are great benefits when babies drink from cups:

- Babies get the opportunities to practice the fine motor skills of holding cups and bringing them to their mouths.

- Sugar from the formula or juice can rot your babies' teeth if they drink from bottles at night or all day long.

- Some babies may get ear infection while lying down and drinking from a bottle. The formula or juice from the bottle staying in the mouth can go to the ear and cause ear infection.

**Q: There are many different types of cups in the market. Which one should my baby use and how should I introduce it?**

A: A cup with a lid and a free flowing spout makes a good choice.

Start with a small amount of water. When your baby has mastered the skills of drinking from a cup, you can start putting breast milk or formula in it.

**Q: Which finger food should I start?**

A: O-shaped cereals, teething crackers, bite-size of soft-cooked vegetables, or fruits (without skin to begin with) are good choices for beginners. As your baby progresses, you can introduce different textures and varieties of foods.

**Q: Should I make my own baby vegetables? I heard that some vegetables might have a harmful substance, i.e. nitrate?**

A: Yes. You can make your own pureed vegetables for your baby.

Nitrates naturally occur in some vegetables, including spinach, beets, green beans, squash, and carrots. The amount of nitrates in these vegetables usually does not cause any harmful effects to older babies unless these foods are contaminated with nitrate polluted water.

American Academy of Pediatric recommends that infants should not eat these foods until after three months of age. Babies younger than three months of age should only have breast milk or formula and should not eat solid foods at all.

**Q: How much juice should I offer to my baby?**

A: Juice is not an essential part of babies' diet. Babies can get the nutrients from eating fresh pureed (or baby) fruits. If you choose to provide juice to your baby, limit the amount to 4-6 ounces a day and serve it in a cup.

Drinking excessive juice is not good for babies. First, drinking too much juice may affect children's appetite for regular meals. Second, calories from excessive juice consumption may cause your child to become overweight or obese.

**Q: My baby is constipated.  What can I do to alleviate the problem?**

A.  Some babies may go for a day or two without a bowel movement. When babies' stools are soft and easily to eliminate, the babies are not constipated. Talk to your baby's doctor, if babies' stools are hard and difficult to eliminate. Many factors can cause constipation:

- The child does not have enough fiber or fluid in the diet.

- The child ignores the signal due to other distractions or anxiety over bowel movements due to prior unpleasant experiences.

- Some medications may cause or worsen constipation.

- Some medical conditions, for example, low muscle tones, may cause stools difficult to eliminate.

Your baby's doctor will help you to figure out the causes and come up with a treatment plan.

Not having enough fiber or liquids in the diet are the most common causes of constipation. If your baby is eating solid foods, the baby's doctor may refer you to a registered dietitian.  A registered dietitian can assess your baby's diet and come up with some practical tips to increase fiber in the diet. It is very important to make sure that your baby is getting enough liquids, while increasing fiber in the diet.

Whole grains, legumes, fruits, and vegetables are good sources of fiber. Legumes such as beans and peas are excellent sources of fiber.  Fruits high in fiber include apricots, peaches, prunes, plums, pears, bananas, strawberries, blueberries, and apples. Vegetables such as peas, spinach, corn, broccoli, green beans, squash, and carrots are also high in fiber.  If you are buying baby foods, read the food labels on the jars to compare the fiber content.

# Chapter 5

# Dietary Recommendations for Children at Different Developmental Stages

In this chapter, we shall cover the recommended food intake for infants and young children, portion sizes, and answers to the frequently asked questions.

A child's growth and development are highly individualized and unique to each child. Many factors, including gender, age, and body size, affect a child's nutritional needs. Talk to your child's doctor if you have concerns about your child's growth and development.

The following are good indicators that your children are getting enough calories and nutrients from the food they eat:

- They eat a wide variety of food.

- They are growing properly with their own growth curves.

## Recommended Food Intake

Parents often wonder the types and the amount of foods to offer to their babies. The dietary recommendations listed below are based on the babies' developmental stages, not based on their chronological age.

## When a baby sits independently

He or she can drink from cups and consume all food groups with the suggested amounts listed in Table 5-1. Most babies reach this developmental milestone at about six months of age.

Table 5-1: The recommended food intake for a baby who sits independently.

| Food Group | Recommended Daily Intake |
|---|---|
| Breast milk or formula | 24 ounces |
| Grains and Cereals | 8 tablespoons or ½ cup |
| Vegetables | 4 tablespoons or ¼ cup |
| Fruits | 4 tablespoons or ¼ cup |
| Meats/Beans | 2 tablespoons or 1 ounce |

# When babies can crawl with their stomachs off the floor

You can offer more vegetables and fruits. They can have ½ cup of fruits and ½ cup of vegetables a day as illustrated in Table 5-2. Most babies reach this developmental stage when they are eight or nine months of age.

Table 5-2: The recommended food intake for a baby who can crawl.

| Food Group | Recommended Daily Intake |
|---|---|
| Breast milk or formula | 24 ounces |
| Grains and Cereals | 8 tablespoons or ½ cup |
| Vegetables | 8 tablespoons or ½ cup |
| Fruits | 8 tablespoons or ½ cup |
| Meats/Beans | 2 tablespoons or 1 ounce |

## When a child can stand up and start walking

It is recommended that you gradually decrease the amount of breast milk or formula that you offer to your baby while increase the amount of fruits, vegetables, and meats/beans. At this developmental stage, children only need two cups of breast milk or formula a day as illustrated in Table 5-3. Many children reach this milestone when they are twelve months of age.

Table 5-3: The recommended intake for a child who can walk.

| Food Group | Recommended Daily Intake |
|---|---|
| Breast milk or formula | 16 ounces or 2 cups |
| Grains and Cereals | 2 ounces |
| Vegetables | 12 tablespoons or ¾ cup |
| Fruits | 16 tablespoons or 1 cup |
| Meats/Beans | 4 tablespoons, ¼ cup or 2 ounces |

## Toddlers

Toddlers can feed themselves with utensils, drink from cups, and consume a wide variety of foods. Table 5-4 illustrates the recommended intake for a toddler.

Table 5-4: The recommended intake for a toddler.

| Food Group | Recommended Daily Intake |
|---|---|
| Dairy/Milk | 2 cups |
| Grains and Cereals | 3-4 ounces |
| Vegetables | 1-1 ½ cups |
| Fruits | 1 –1 ½ cups |
| Meats/Fish/Beans | 2 ounces – 3 ounces |

# Food Portion Sizes

**Milk and dairy products:** They are good sources of protein, calcium, potassium, and vitamin D. They are important for babies' bone growth and development. One serving of dairy products equals:

> 1 cup of milk or soymilk
>
> 1 cup of yogurt
>
> 1 ½ ounces of cheese
>
> ½ cup of cottage cheese (Cottage cheese has higher protein and lower calcium contents compared to other dairy products.)

Yogurt, like other dairy products, offers many essential nutrients. In addition, yogurt contains active culture known as probiotics.  Probiotics (good bacteria) can help maintain a healthy digestive gut, boost our bodies' abilities to fight germs, and may reduce eczema in young children.

**Grains and cereals**: They contain energy and nutrients for our body. Whole grains and cereals are also good sources of dietary fibers. Most grains and cereals are fortified with B vitamins, such as thiamin, niacin, riboflavin, and folic acid. In addition, some of the breakfast cereals are enriched with minerals, like iron. One serving or one ounce of grains/cereals equals:

> one slice of bread
>
> ½ cup of pasta
>
> ½ cup of cooked rice
>
> ½ cup of cooked cereals
>
> ¾ - 1 cup of breakfast cereal
>
> one tortilla (6 inches across)

3 Graham crackers

6 saltine crackers

**Vegetables:** Vegetables are an important part of a healthy diet. They are excellent sources of dietary fibers and contain many essential vitamins and minerals, including folate, vitamin A, vitamin C, vitamin K, magnesium, and potassium. One cup of vegetables equals:

1 cup of raw vegetables

½ cup of cooked vegetables (Most leafy vegetables will shrink when cooked.)

If you have doubts whether young children can handle the sizes or the textures of some vegetables, you may:

- cook down the vegetables (Cooking makes the texture softer);

- put them in the grinder and make pureed vegetables; or

- chop the vegetables into smaller pieces.

**Fruits:** Fruits provide nutrients vital for health, with dietary fiber, vitamins, and minerals. Most fruits are naturally low in fat and sodium. Fruits make great snacks and can be part of healthy meals. One cup of fruit equals:

one small size apple, orange, or peach

½ cup of applesauce

½ cup of canned fruits

1 cup of melon or papaya cubes

½ bananas

½ cup of juice

2 tablespoons of raisins

**Meats, fish, and beans:** They are rich in protein, zinc, and iron essential for babies' growth and development. Fish for example, salmon and tuna, contains omega-3 fatty acids, including eicosapentaenoic acid (EPA) and docosahexaenoic acid (DHA). EPA and DHA are beneficial to the baby's brain and eye development. Beans, including kidney beans, pinto beans, black beans, lima beans, and lentils are  excellent sources of dietary fiber, potassium, and folate. One serving or one ounce of meat/fish/beans equals:

1 egg

¼ cup of cooked beans

1 slice of deli meats or 1 ounce of meats

3 ounces of Tofu

# Frequently Asked Questions and Answers

**Q: Why does my child need to have iron-rich foods?**

A: Iron is an essential nutrient that helps children learn and grow.  Iron is important for keeping our blood and brain healthy. Good sources of iron include iron fortified cereals, meats, and green leafy vegetables.

**Q: My baby (or child) fails to gain weight. What should I do?**

A:  Every child's growth pattern is different and unique.  It is normal for a child to eat a lot during growth spurts and then decrease his or her appetite and food intake dramatically when growth rate slows down.

Talk to your child's doctor if you have concerns and questions about your child's growth pattern. The doctor can help you figure out the causes and come up with a treatment plan. The doctor may also refer you to see a registered dietitian who can provide you with practical tips to increase calories in your child's diet.

If your baby can eat solid foods, you may consider increasing calories in your child's diet in the following ways:

o   Offer higher caloric dense food such as yogurt or pudding as a snack.

o   Add a teaspoon of corn oil or vegetable oil to 4 ounces of baby vegetables or meats. Adding olive oil or flax seed oil to solid foods can also help if your children like them.

o   Avocado is high in calories and contains many nutrients. It can be a good snack by itself, mashed and mixed with other foods, or served as dips or spreads.

o   For older babies (nine months or older) and young children, consider adding wheat germs to a variety of foods. Wheat germs can be found in the cereal aisle inside a grocery store. One tablespoon of Wheat germs provides 25 calories and many nutrients.

o   For children (12 months or older), making delicious high calorie milk shakes is a good option.  You can experiment with adding ice cream and a variety of fruits to milk and then mix them in a blender. This makes delicious milk shakes with extra calories and nutrients without much increase in volume.

o   For children (12 months or older), another option is adding one packet of carnation instant breakfast to 1 cup of whole milk. One packet of carnation instant breakfast provides 130 calories.

You can find carnation instant breakfast in the cereal or milk powder aisle inside a grocery store.

Many babies and toddlers will start gaining weight when they get an extra 100 calories from the food they eat in their daily diet.

# Chapter 6

## Building Healthy Eating Habits in Early Childhood Provides Life-Long Benefits

In this chapter, we shall discuss healthy eating habits, family meals, and strategies to help your child build healthy eating habits.

Many lifetime habits are formed in early childhood. It is important to do it right from the start. Eating healthy foods will provide energy and nutrients that children need for their growth and development.

## Healthy Eating Habits

Healthy eating habits are good for everyone in the family:

- Eat plenty of wholesome foods – fresh fruits, vegetables, and whole grains. Buy fruits and vegetables in season, they are fresh and more affordable.

- Reduce consumption of saturated fats and trans fats. Saturated fats are found in meats such as beef, pork, and chicken. Trans fats are usually found in processed food. Read the food label to learn more about the amount of saturated fats and trans fats in the products you buy.

- Consume less of sugar and sweets.  Excessive sugary foods replace more nutritious foods, increase the risk for tooth decay, affect blood sugar level, may cause mood swings, and digestive problems. Read and compare the nutrition facts on the packages and choose the product with less sugar.

- Watch out for salt and salty foods. Salt enhances flavor in food. It induces our desire to eat more often and in larger quantities. Many food companies add salt to bread to improve the taste. One slice of bread may contain 10% of sodium daily intake for an adult. Read and compare the nutrition facts on the packages and choose the product with less salt.

- Choose fresh wholesome food over highly processed foods. Many natural nutrients in these foods are destroyed during food processing. Second, food companies add sugar, fat, food flavorings, and colorings to make food look more appealing, more palatable, and easier to eat.  When children eat these highly processed foods, they tend to eat more than what their bodies' need. Third, too much sugar or additives may cause mood swing or other adverse symptoms. Read the food label and the ingredient list and choose wisely.

- Drink plenty of water instead of sweet beverages, including soda and juice drinks. Americans consume large quantities of sweet beverages. In fact, sweet beverages have become the main source of added sugar for many children.

- Active culture can be a good thing for your children. Yogurt or soy yogurt contains active culture. Good bacteria in the active culture can help our bodies build and maintain healthy gut for food absorption, digestion, and metabolism.

# Family Meals

Many American families do not sit and eat together due to busy schedules. They often forego the food preparation, purchase packaged and ready-to-eat products, and gobble them down in 5 – 10 minutes. Poor eating habits like these have caused many chronic diseases and health problems in addition to overweight and obesity. It is time for us to change this and we can start with our own family.

Studies have shown that there are many benefits to children when family members eat together:

- Children with family meals eat healthier food. Studies have shown that when people eat together, they eat more vegetables and less processed food.

- Family meals provide opportunities for children to learn social behaviors, table manners, and proper dining etiquette. Start with small steps and encourage children to:

    o   Listen and take turns talking.

    o   Turn off TV during meal times.

    o   Get a small serving first, when needed, have a second serving.

    o   Decide how much they are going to eat.

- Studies have shown that children eat together as a family is happier and even doing better at school.

# Frequently Asked Questions and Answers

**Q: My baby and young children do not like vegetables. What can I do?**

A: Every child is different. Many options are available. To encourage your children to eat a variety of foods, you can:

- **Have fun introducing new vegetables**. Engage them in food shopping and preparation as much as possible. They are more likely to eat the food that they help pick and prepare. If time and space allow, grow your own vegetable garden. It is fun for kids to be involved in growing their own vegetables. Children are more likely to try the food they grow.

- **Introduce pureed vegetables before pureed fruits**. Generally speaking, vegetables are not as sweet as fruits. Some babies are willing to eat a variety of foods while others may need more exposure before they try new foods. Be patient and continue to offer vegetables.

- **Introduce new food when your toddler is hungry.** This increases the chance that he or she eats it.

- **Offer only one new food at a time.** Children can be overwhelmed by too many new food items at one time.

- **Serve a variety of easy to manage foods.** Pay attention to food temperature and textures. Make sure that the food temperature and textures are easy for your young child to manage. Many children prefer foods that do not require a lot of chewing even if they can handle the texture. Sometimes, you can soften the texture by cooking it longer.

- **Do not worry if your child decides to eat only certain foods for a few days.** Studies have shown that when healthy food choices are available, the majority of healthy babies and toddlers will self-regulate their food intake and get enough calories and nutrients.

- **Do not bribe your child to eat.** This may create a power struggle if your child refuses to eat.

- **Make sure your child eats at the table or in the highchair.** It is not a good idea to allow them to graze all over the place.

- **Eliminate as many distractions as possible at mealtimes.** For example, turn off the TV during mealtimes.

- **Limit the choices.** If you prefer giving choices, limit the choices to two. Some children may reject foods so they feel that they have some control.

- **Avoid big portion sizes and keep it simple.** Too many food items with large portion sizes on a plate may be too overwhelming for some children.

- **Stay calm during mealtimes.** Pushing your child to eat has adverse impact. It gives him or her negative attention and increases pickiness. Worrying only makes things worse. If your child refuses to try a new food, offer it again few days later with a small amount. For some babies, it might take more than ten exposures before they eat something new to them. Children are more likely to try new food in a relaxed and pleasant environment.

**Q: Should I have a mealtime schedule for my baby?**

A: When your baby is old enough for solid foods, it is helpful to form a routine for meals and snacks. For many older babies and toddlers, three meals and three snacks a day will meet their needs. It is not a good idea to allow your child to graze all day even if you are concerned about his or her weight gain. Spacing between meals and snacks for 2-3 hours allows the children to feel hungry and eat to their satiety.

**Q: How do I prevent my child from having tooth decay?**

A: Baby teeth usually appear after six months of age. Baby teeth help children chew and speak and also hold space in the jaws for permanent teeth that are growing under the gums. It is very important to keep them healthy:

- Do not allow your child taking a bottle to bed.

- Do not put juice in a bottle. When your child is old enough for juice, introduce juice in a cup and limit it to four ounces a day.

- Avoid sweet beverages. Sugar contents in these beverages are substrates for bacteria in the mouths to produce acids. Acids can cause dental cavities.

- Brush your baby's teeth with water twice a day to keep them clean. Toddlers may cooperate with brushing teeth. Children at two years of age or older can use fluoride toothpaste.

- Take your baby to the dentist before your baby's first birthday.

**Q: Can I start my child on a vegan diet?**

A: Yes. Vegan diets can provide adequate energy and nutrients for your child's growing needs if well planned.

People on a vegan diet only consume food from plant sources. They do not eat dairy products, eggs, and meats. The key to a healthy vegan diet is to consume a wide variety of food. Like other children, children on vegan diet can self-regulate their food intake to meet their needs.

When a child is on a vegan diet, it is important for parents to pay attention to the following nutrients:

### Protein

Protein is one of the three main sources of body energy. Protein is needed for the growth and health of a child. One gram of protein provides four calories. Good sources of protein in a vegan diet include:

- Beans, lentils, peas, and wheat-based (gluten) meat analogs, for example, veggie burgers, are good sources of protein.

- Tofu is a soybean product and comes in different consistencies: pudding, soft, regular, and firm. It has a plain taste. You can add it to stir fries, marinated it the way you like it, use it to replace meats, and even make deserts with it.

When your children are old enough to handle nuts without the risk of choking, be sure to include nuts into their diet. Nuts are rich in protein and good fat.

### Iron

Iron is an essential nutrient needed for blood cells and other body functions. Infant cereals, iron fortified breakfast cereals, dried fruits, and food cooked in cast iron pans are good sources of iron.

## Calcium

Calcium is a mineral needed for bone growth and for our general health.

Breast milk, soy infant formula, soybean milk, soy yogurt, and calcium fortified juice are rich in calcium.

Food with active culture such as soy yogurt will provide calcium as well as other nutrients. It can offer many health benefits to your child.

## Zinc

Zinc is a mineral that is needed for muscles and our health. Foods rich in protein are also rich in zinc. Beans, lentils, peas, wheat-based (gluten) meat analogs, soybean products, and veggie burgers are good sources of zinc.

In addition, when your child is nine months or older, you can start offering wheat germs. They are also rich in zinc.

## Riboflavin (Vitamin B2)

Riboflavin is a water-soluble vitamin and is needed for body metabolism. Whole grains, fortified soybean milk, legumes, and fortified breakfast cereals are good sources of riboflavin.

## Vitamin B12

Vitamin B12 is a water-soluble vitamin needed for red blood cell and body metabolism. A lot of products, for example, soybean milk, breakfast cereals, and meat analogs, are fortified with vitamin B12. Read the nutrition facts on the food labels and choose the products fortified with vitamin B12.

## Vitamin D

Vitamin D is a fat-soluble vitamin needed for healthy bones. Good sources of vitamin D in a vegan diet include vitamin D fortified soy milk, vitamin D fortified orange juice, and other products fortified with vitamin D.

# Glossary

**Allergen:** A substance that causes an allergic reaction.

**Bacteria:** Single-celled microbes. Some are good for our health such as the ones in yogurt. Other bacteria are potentially disease causing.

**Body Mass Index (BMI):** An index of relating a person's weight to height.

**Calories:** Units of energy measurements in food.

**Dietary fiber:** The non-digestible carbohydrates found in foods such as whole grain products, fruits, vegetables, and legumes. Dietary fibers promote bowel movement and may decrease your risk for some diseases.

**Dietitian:** A healthcare professional who specializes in food and nutrition.

**Epidemic:** A health problem that affects many people at the same time.

**Fine motor skills:** The skill and ability to use the smaller muscles in the arms, hands, and fingers such as using a spoon to eat.

**Lanolin:** Grease (wax) secreted from wool-bearing animals, such as sheep.

**Nutrition fact label:** A label on food packages that gives the serving size, servings per container, calories per serving, and other information on nutrients.

**Nutrients:** They are found in food. The body uses nutrients to grow, function, and stay alive. The major classes of nutrients include water, proteins, carbohydrates, fats, minerals, and vitamins.

**Prebiotics:** Non-digestible food ingredients that stimulate the growth and/or activity of good bacteria (Probiotics) in the digestive system.

**Probiotics:** Live microorganisms beneficial to the host.

**Protein:** One of the three major nutrients in food that provides us with energy. Protein is needed for our bodies to build or repair muscles and organs. Protein is found in foods mainly from milk and meat/bean groups.

**Trans fats:** Types of fats that have been manufactured by adding hydrogen bonds to unsaturated fats. These fats are often referred to as "hydrogenated fats" or "partially hydrogenated fats" on the ingredient list.

**Vitamins:** Nutrients found in food; needed in small amounts for us to be healthy and function well.

**Vitamin D**: A fat-soluble vitamin that is important for bone health and bone metabolism.

# Resources

- Active Bodies Active Mind. http://depts.washington.edu/tvhealth/index.htm

- American Academy of Pediatrics: Guide to Your Child's Nutrition.

- Academy of Nutrition and Dietetics. http://www.eatright.org

- Growth Charts. http://www.cdc.gov/growthcharts/who_charts.htm

- La Leche League. http://www.llli.org/

- Pediatrics. http://pediatrics.aappublications.org/

- The Food Allergy & Anaphylaxis Network. http://www.foodallergy.org/

- http://www.nutrition.gov

# Author

Yuchi Yang is a registered dietitian with over twenty years of professional experience. She is a graduate of Taipei Medical College in Nutrition and holds a master degree from the University of Connecticut in Nutritional Science. She had her nutrition internship specialized in children with developmental disabilities with the University of California, Los Angeles.

Yuchi enjoys working with children and families to address their nutritional concerns. Yuchi was a nutrition consultant with the Children with Special Health Care Needs Program with the Department of Health in the state of Washington. She worked as a clinical dietitian at Children's Hospital, Los Angeles. She was a supervisory nutritionist with the Women, Infants, and Children (WIC) Program in San Mateo County in the state of California. She was a WIC nutritionist in Watts Health Foundation in Los Angeles and a WIC dietitian in Gouverneur Hospital in New York City. She is also the founder of American Nutrition Counseling, LLC located in Issaquah, Washington (http://www.anutritioncounseling.com).

# Disclaimer

The information provided in this book is general recommendations for healthy babies and toddlers. The information provided in this book should not be used for diagnosing purposes or be substituted for medical advice. As with any new or ongoing treatment, always consult with your doctor before beginning any new treatment.

The author provides resources and links for your information only. The author is not responsible for the products or contents provided in these web sites.

Made in the USA
Lexington, KY
27 March 2012